DMSO: THE REVOLUTIONARY NATURE'S WONDER DRUG.

DMSO Therapy for: Emergency Medicine, Multiple Sclerosis, Amyloidosis, Burn Injuries, Headaches, Scleroderma, Pains, Arthritis, Lupus, Athletic Injuries, Brain Injuries, Alzheimer's And Other Dementia, Tooth & Gum Disease, Shingles & Herpes, Cirrhosis of the Liver, Diabetes, Carpal Tunnel Syndrome, Digestive Problems, Hair And Scalp Problems, Fungus Infection, Inflammatory Disease, Interstitial Cystitis, Asthmatic Condition, And Stroke.

By

Dr. Stephanie Dean.

Table of Contents.

CHAPTER 1

INTRODUCTION TO DMSO.

Dimethyl sulfoxide, popularly known as DMSO, has been described by many people particularly those who have used it as a true miracle medicine. This product (DMSO) has been used by medical experts to treat several medical conditions that alter the health and well-being of patients around the globe. A combination of DMSO with other medications or its singular usage has been proven to be a useful treatment for virtually all known ailments.

♣ Definition of DMSO.

DMSO is defined as a natural chemical compound, a by-product of trees gotten through the process of paper manufacturing. It is basically made of two groups of Methyl (CH_3), and sulfur, alongside oxygen atoms.

♣ <u>Functions Of DMSO.</u>

- **<u>Normalize Immune System:</u>** Normalizing immunity is another good function of DMSO as it makes it easier to treat auto-immune related diseases and further enables the natural immune system to ward off diverse infectious and transferrable diseases.

- **<u>Skin Permeability:</u>** DMSO has the capacity to pass through the skin and other cellular tissues of the body. DMSO, among other products, can cross through the blood-brain barrier while conveniently taking in other products that cannot cross the blood barrier thereby making

DMSO a valuable product in treating most brain problems.

- **<u>Vasodilator/Vasorelaxation:</u>** Vasodilator simply means widening of the blood vessels thereby aiding the free flow of blood. DMSO helps increase easy blood flow to damaged areas of the body. Sometimes, DMSO tends to treat other ailments in the body besides the actual ailment that the product is being used for.

♣ <u>DMSO As An Emergency Medicine.</u>

Over the years, DMSO as an alternative medicine has proven to be very effective in treating a wide range of ailments without any negative contrary effects. This has made it a must-have medication in any emergency room, ambulance, or paramedic unit, and for trained first aiders with adequate instructional guides on how to use this medicine.

Several elements in DMSO make it a wanted healing agent in treating accident victims with sudden serious ailments like stroke or cardiac arrest hence, there have not been much arguments on the use of solution (DMSO) in emergencies. DMSO helps elevate edema (swollen feed), it is an anti-inflammatory medication, it helps enhance oxygen supply, and also protects the body cells from any mechanical damage that may occur due to its free radical scavenger nature. The whole essence of having DMSO as part of our emergency drug is to prevent any progressive damage that may occur as a result of injuries sustained by the individual and topical application of DMSO to the injured area is often the first treatment method followed by maybe intravenous method or the oral method.

There have been several testimonies of how DMSO was used as an emergency medication on patients whose health cases have been concluded closed (no hope for their survival) and they got healed at the end with amazing recovery speed and without any scars or trace of them being ever sick. I believe as time progresses, DMSO as a therapy will be allowed to strive in the medical world as a go-to drug in emergencies; particularly the topical application method which is generally the simplest method that can be learned by anyone irrespective of age and profession with proper training and use safely at our conveniences because DMSO seems not be known globally.

CHAPTER 2

HISTORY OF DMSO.

DMSO was made known by a Russian chemist in 1866 and for several years, this product remained ignored by all. Industrial chemists began investigating this natural product (DMSO) by late 1940, to know its capabilities and the positive benefits it can offer. For over eighty years DMSO was basically ignored. This came about when there was the need for better-quality solvents and there was interest in the use of waste products obtained from trees. DMSO development commenced commercially in the 1950s by an American paper manufacturing organization which brought the knowledge of DMSO into the limelight. Before the advent of DMSO, there were no positive methods to preserve transplanted organs without forming ice crystals that often kill the tissue until DMSO's anti-freezing potential came into reality.

DMSO has been described by experts as a new medical principle; a substance that is strange to medical sciences, with a mode of action that is mysterious to people but used to treat sicknesses that have been considered incurable. It is often difficult to carry out double-masked tests on DMSO because of its unique odor but it is possible to get studies that involve comparing DMSO alongside present medication. For instance, if a particular disease has a mortality rate of 80% at a certain level in a year without the use of DMSO therapy and a 10% mortality rate for those treated with DMSO therapy, this shows the positive effectiveness of DMSO as a healing agent.

♣ <u>Toxicity In DMSO.</u>

DMSO has long been seen and believed to be one of, if not the safest products ever used in medicine when it comes to treating several ailments. No case of death or severe injury has been recorded via its usage by different individuals over the years across the globe. Although the toxic effect (changes in animal's eye lens) recorded as a result of using this medicine on some animals (dogs, pigs, and rabbits) due to the massive dose of the medicine given to these animals gave a bad review of this amazing healing agent. Though it didn't have any negative effect when used on humans and other animals like donkeys, but the initial negative review given to the medicine never ceased to spread until another toxicology study was carried out at Vacaville California between the years 1967 and

1968, where DMSO was proven to be a totally safe medicine void of any negative toxic effect. These studies were done by topically applying an 80% concentration of DMSO solution on the skin using a rate of 1gm per kg of the individual's body weight daily between 3-30 30-minute intervals. The researchers who carried out this study ensured that individuals used for this experiment were void of any health impediments either physically, mentally, or emotionally. The studies were carried out at different time intervals (14 days, 2 weeks after, and 4 weeks after). At the end of the experiment, no negative reactions were recorded though there was scaling and dryness in the skin which later returned to normal within a few weeks after the treatment.

This result brought about the final conclusion on the safety of DMSO therapy for humans and other animals. From the studies, it was observed that the changes observed in some animal's eye lenses did not occur in humans even with higher doses.

CHAPTER 3

DMSO THERAPY FOR SOME AILMENTS.

♣ Amyloidosis.

Amyloidosis is a disease that results from a build-up of amyloid proteins in different tissues of the body and its symptoms basically depend on the organ(s) affected. The disease is often difficult to diagnose particularly at its early stage hence leaving so many of its victims undiagnosed. Because it can affect many internal organs of the body, its symptoms are usually similar to other conditions; this makes one suspect other ailment.

Amyloidosis disease is classified basically into two categories;

- Localized form and
- Systemic form.

The localized form of Amyloidosis majorly affects a particular organ or part of the body without damaging the remaining parts of the body system. Common conditions associated with this category include; type 2 diabetes (where amyloid protein develops in the pancreas) and Alzheimer's (where the brain experiences the build-up of amyloid protein).

Unlike the localized Amyloidosis which affects only a part of the body, the Systemic amyloidosis has the capacity to cause damage to any part/organs of the body. Different organs of the body (heart, respiratory tract, spleen, gastrointestinal tract, etc.) are often involved in this category and may result in death due to the presence of various toxic activities in the affected organs.

Several studies have shown the effective impact of DMSO therapy on Amyloidosis disease without any adverse effects on its usage. For instance, a case study of some mice that were induced with Amyloidosis; some were treated with DMSO while some were left untreated; these mice were studied for 60 days before they were killed and an autopsy was carried out on them. Their urine while further tested and it was observed that the urine of the DMSO-treated mice showed traces of broken amyloid fluids which came as a result of the DMSO treatment administered with their livers totally devoid of amyloid deposits while the livers of the control mice (mice without DMSO treatment) have amyloids stock up in them.

With the above illustration in mind, one would agree that DMSO is a good option treatment for

Amyloidosis. *Note: DMSO should not be administered solely but combined with other medications to help those medications work efficiently.*

♣ <u>Burn Injuries.</u>

Lotions with DMSO solution in their contents have proven to be very potent in the treatment of burn injuries. Burn injuries are often very painful and fatal irrespective of their severity. Aside the damage this injury causes to the affected tissue, the area(s) affected can also get infected. With the help of DMSO solution contained in lotions particularly a mixture of DMSO solution and aloe vera, blisters formation among many other after-effects of burn injuries are prevented, and a quick recovery process.

<u>Treatment Procedure.</u>

<u>Topically:</u> Mix a 50% concentration of DMSO solution with 50% solution of aloe vera and apply it to the affected area immediately after the accident takes place. Administer the same treatment after one hour and 3 hours after the second application.

Apply the mixture every 8 hours for the next two days after the incident.

♣ <u>DMSO Therapy For Headaches.</u>

Headaches are one ailment that affects everyone at some point in our lives. Headaches are of various types and nearly half of the world population experiences at least one type of headache or the other each month. It often results from muscle tremors around the neck region or variations in blood vessels that goes into the individual's head or the way our body systems react to emotional stresses that we encounter daily. Oftentimes, aspirin is usually the first treatment most headache patients go for but the results differ particularly in migraine headache cases (it barely responds to aspirin treatment).

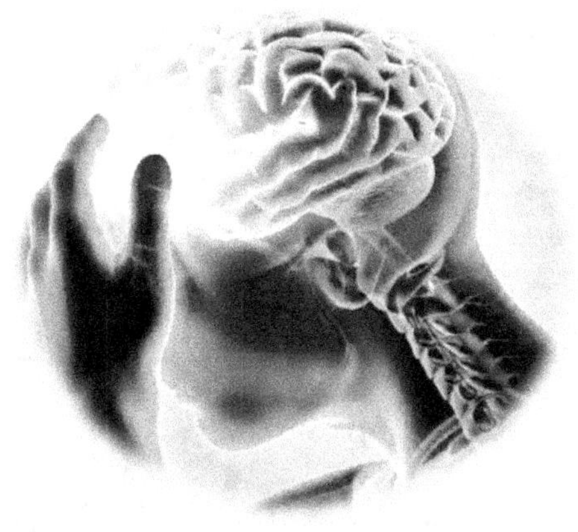

DMSO has over the years been used to treat this ailment with minimal or no side effects compared to other conventional treatments used years back. From observation, if migraine headaches are treated in their early developmental stages, it is easier to reverse the condition with the help of a DMSO solution. Therefore, administering the solution (DMSO) to the patient early enough is very important to their recovery process.

Treatment Procedure.

The regular DMSO treatment for headaches is;

<u>Topically:</u> By massaging DMSO solution to the patient's neck and head regularly.

<u>Orally:</u> Let the patient drink a teaspoon of DMSO solution mixed in a cup of juice or water daily.

♣ Pains.

Pain is a signal to the body system that something is wrong and the ability of DMSO to reduce pain is one major benefit that makes it outstanding amongst other alternative medicines. Pain appears in diverse forms which often occurs as a result of accidents either domestic or otherwise which often renders its victims immobile for some time. Pain warns the patient of potential danger that can cause harm or damage to the body.

Even though DMSO can reduce pain, it's not meant to take the place of a medical expert, hence finding the root cause of any pain and getting the right advice from a physician is paramount. Although two different persons can show the same symptoms for the same ailment but different severity levels particularly back pains.

<u>Treatment Procedure.</u>

Topically apply lotion contained with a 90% concentration of DMSO solution to the affected area twice daily until relief is achieved and proper mobility is restored.

♣ <u>Phantom Pain With DMSO Therapy.</u>

Phantom pain is one serious pain that patient suffers today. It is a pain that affects one lost part of the body (an amputated leg or arm). It comes in the form of a tingling or burning sensation, and severe or dull pain in part of the entire missing part of the body.

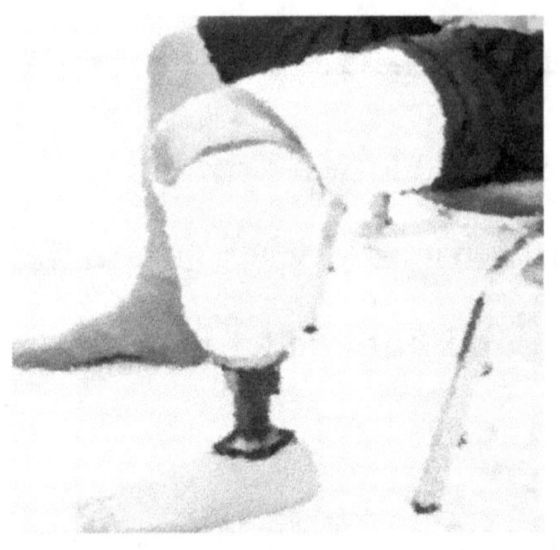

The victim might feel numbness in that missing part in most cases. Sometimes, this type of pain is usually difficult to treat but with DMSO, relief is very certain.

Treatment Procedure.

Get a lotion contained in a mixture of DMSO solution, aloe vera juice, and capsicum pepper and apply to the affected area (amputated area) twice daily for 3 months or till total recovery is achieved.

CHAPTER 4
DMSO THERAPY FOR ARTHRITIS CONDITION.

According to reports from the Arthritis Foundation, several persons (more than 20 million) suffer from arthritis impairment. This disease can be mild most times with minor pains while in most cases, it can be severely painful leading to immobility in the sufferer. Arthritis is one of the leading causes of disabilities in people aged 60 and above. This disease does not have a particular medication; medical experts only use usual medications like painkillers, cortisone, aspirin, and an anti-inflammatory drug (non-steroidal) which only lessen the pain and not put a permanent stop to this ailment. Although these medicines reduce the pain from the ailment, but can be very dangerous to the patient's health when taken for a long duration particularly the non-steroidal anti-inflammatory medication that affects joints, blocks the enzyme inflammatory-producing compounds, and also restrains the action of the enzymes that produces cartilage in the body system.

To date, DMSO has been proven by medical experts and even arthritis patients who have received DMSO treatment, to be the best medical solution for any form of arthritis ailment. It can be used as a sole treatment or in combination with other medications like glucosamine sulfate or MSM (Methylsulfonylmethane). DMSO can be applied topically (massage it on the affected area), via injection, or orally.

♣ <u>Effects Of DMSO Solution On Arthritis.</u>

DMSO has several positive effects on arthritis conditions without any side reaction, ranging from;

1. Reducing pains and cramps around the affected joints

2. Enhances blood flow and brings in the necessary amount of nutrients required around the affected area.

3. It provides natural sulfur to the affected area.

4. Reduce inflammation of joints

5. It inhibits the development of free radicals (unstable atoms with the ability to cause damage to cells in the body).

<u>Treatment Procedure.</u>

- <u>Topically</u> – Apply 90% concentration solution of DMSO to the affected area daily.

- <u>Orally</u> – Drink a teaspoon of 90% solution of the product (DMSO) in 4 ounces of any favorite juice or water daily.

- <u>Intravenously</u> – Combine 5% concentration of DMSO solution with magnesium sulfate, vitamin C, and B complex, inject it into the patient twice a week for 5 weeks, and then reduce it to once a month for a period of 1 year and 6 months. The intravenous method of application helps reduce free radical effects in the body.

Note.....DMSO medication should not be taken without proper medical supervision.

CHAPTER 5

DMSO THERAPY FOR ATHLETIC INJURIES.

Over the years, great success has been recorded in the treatment of Athletic injuries using DMSO solution. Athletic injuries are not mainly those injuries that require surgical procedures, bone settings, or traumatic conditions that need immediate medical attention. They include those common injuries that brood gradually or as a result of intense workouts or sports activities. Most times there might not be accidents but there will be an injury that emanates from the constant pounding, and regular use of the muscles, tendons, and joints, etc., endurance activities like marathons can result in injuries on the hip, knee, and other body parts that may show up immediately or after some days or months of engaging in those activities. However, these damages mentioned, can be reduced or cleared off by the regular use of DMSO solution; topically apply it on your legs or take a teaspoonful of the solution mixed in a glass of juice or water orally before or immediately after any major workouts help reduce inflammation that may occur as a result of the exercise activities.

Being available to compete in any athletic activities, is the most important thing to any athlete out there, and any serious injury that renders a professional athlete unfit to compete leads to loss to such athlete financially. In the real sense, no athlete wants to be in the group while others whom he competes with, use DMSO. Though DMSO as a solution is not prohibited nor is it a performance-enhancing medication, many athletes find it difficult to tell others what they use as a medication to relieve pains or reduce downtime experiences. DMSO is one medicine that should be known by every athlete because of its numerous benefits. Some athletes such as footballers and boxers suffer brain damage due to physical contact while playing football games or constant hitting on the head during boxing. However, with the help of DMSO's regular usage after each activity, this brain damage tends to reduce and even go unnoticed by the individual while those with obvious signs of head injury can take the intravenous (injection) DMSO solution to reduce possible long-term damage to the victim.

Injuries during athletic activities are inevitable, but measures should be put in place to limit these injuries as well as quick and complete recovery measures for injured athletes to prevent disabilities.

Treatment Procedure.

- <u>Topical:</u> Simple massaging of DMSO solution on the head for brain injuries or to prevent its symptoms.

- <u>Oral:</u> Drink a teaspoon of DMSO mixed with any fruit juice of your choice or water before or after any activity.

- <u>Intravenous:</u> DMSO solution can be injected.

- With other drugs: DMSO solution can be combined with other products and given to the individual to enhance the resultant effect.

CHAPTER 6

DMSO THERAPY FOR BRAIN-RELATED AILMENTS.

♣ Brain Injuries.

Brain injuries often occur as a result of accidents from automobiles, industries, falls from heights, or even traumas. These injuries are often very difficult to treat using regular modern medicines and can lead to several other damages that involve nerve injury, free radical formation, edema, decreased blood flow, and a lack of oxygen. In head or brain injury, much of the permanent damage is caused by a reduction of blood flow into the brain. Reduction in blood flow can lead to lack of oxygen and nutrient deficiency in the brain tissue. If this lasts for a significant period, part or all of the brain can be damaged or killed. The final result can be the death of the patient. Another cause of death or disability in head injuries is an accumulation of blood that compresses the brain.

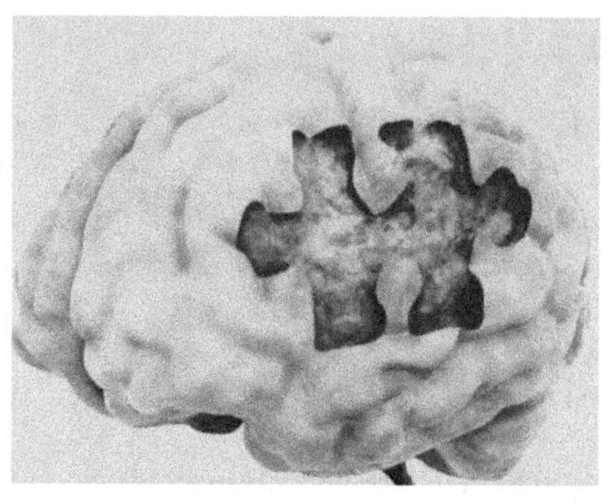

The unique properties of DMSO make it the most useful agent known for treating severe head injuries. DMSO treatment should be started as soon as possible after the injury. There is no definite time limit. Generally, the best results are obtained if treatment is started in the first few minutes after the injury as delay in treatment can result to permanent damage because the brain tissue is delicate and can depreciate swiftly if it's oxygen starved. The use of DMSO which results in better blood flow can help the vascular system remove this excess blood from the cranial cavity. Water can also accumulate in the brain causing pressure on vital parts of the brain. DMSO is the best product available to remove this excess water.

When treatment is delayed certain brain functions can be destroyed permanently or the patient can die. There have been no harmful side effects, and the proper use of DMSO could save the lives of many patients with severe head injuries.

Treatment Procedure.

The normal DMSO treatment for any chronic head injury is basically by the intravenous slow drip application but before the arrival of the intravenous treatment, topical application of

DMSO solution on the head of the victim should be given.

Intravenous treatment: Give 5gms per kg of the patient's body weight for about 24-hours. Then reduce the dosage to about 2-3gms per kg of the patient's body weight after the initial 24 hours. This will help increase blood flow to the brain region.

♣ Alzheimer's And Other Dementia.

Dementia and Alzheimer like every other chronic ailment have increasingly become a major concern to the health of the general population as time goes by. As one advances in age, blood circulation often reduces further resulting in a lack of oxygen and nutrient supplies to the brain system. However, with the help of DMSO solution, this problem can be avoided by helping the various neurons of the brain communicate effectively thereby enabling the individual to retain his/her mental stability even at an advanced age. The ability of DMSO to effectively treat patients with Alzheimer's makes it an important product due to its capacity to melt off amyloids (a protein that is present in the lesion of an Alzheimer's patient's brain).

From research carried out on patients with Alzheimer who were treated with DMSO solution along with regular examination for a period of 9 months. From the regular examinations, it was observed that improvements were recorded within 3 months of this treatment and became more visible after 6 months of using this treatment (DMSO). The improvements were obtained from the neurological tests carried out which show great improvement in the patient's memory, and concentration level alongside their communication skills.

Looking at the above illustration, one would agree that DMSO is a good product for the treatment of brain-related issues (Alzheimer and dementia), and the treatment should be applied immediately after the problem becomes noticeable in any patient because it is often very difficult to reverse the situation once the ailment gets to an advanced stage.

♣ <u>**DMSO Therapy For Mental Illness**</u>

DMSO has over the years been used in treating several mental health cases in patients such as obsessive-compulsive neurosis patients, alcohol-related psychoses, etc.

Studies carried out on the use of DMSO in treating mental prove its effectiveness. These studies were carried out using about 42-patients. These patients were grouped into different categories by level of ailment similarities. These patients were removed from all previous medication a week before DMSO treatment was introduced. Following the treatment procedure, it was shown from the studies that DMSO had a positive recovery effect on mental ailments as the patients felt relief at all points with a faster response to DMSO treatment compared to the conventional treatment that they were been given. With various testimonies on the positive effect of the unique drug (DMSO) in treating several ailments, it has become imperative to have this product in mental hospitals/institutions with a proper user guide to help those mentally ill patients without hope of recovery regain sanity, balance and live a productive life going forward.

Treatment Procedure.

Give 50% to 80% concentration of DMSO solution in a 5-ml intramuscular injection to the patient 2-3 times daily. For very disturbed patients, 5 of the injections can be administered a day. For patients with mild effects, administer just 50% concentration of DMSO solution in a 5ml intramuscular injection.

CHAPTER 7

DMSO THERAPY FOR CANCEROUS AILMENTS.

Over the years, DMSO has been used to treat cancer patients with maximum success level. Several healing properties contained in DMSO solution make it a potent force that should be reckoned with in the treatment of cancer. DMSO is a free radical scavenger as well as a powerful cleansing agent; these qualities give it the ability to penetrate any tissue and cells of the body alone or while carrying other medications alongside. DMSO can be used solely to treat cancer (it is an anti-cancer of its own) or in combination with other anti-cancer medicines.

<u>Treatment Procedure.</u>

<u>Intravenously:</u> **1st Dose:** Administer 4-5mg per kg of the patient's body weight daily till about 3 to 4gms has been given to the patient (without any visible adverse side effects).

<u>2nd Dose:</u> Give a 12-15-day space after the 1st dose and administer another dosage of the same measurement with the 1st dose till another 3-4gms is achieved. This 2nd cycle often depends largely on the patient's general condition and reduction of the cancer ailment.

<u>Life story:</u>

Research carried out on cancer disease revealed the effective treatment of cancer, using DMSO solution in combination with other cancer medications such as amino acid and cyclophosphamide. About 65 cancer patients who were classified to be incurable because they had been treated previously using conventional medications with no positive outcome (due to the toxic effect of medical) were tried with DMSO solution. The cyclophosphamide was melted in a DMSO solution and administered to the patient. There was a maximum decrease in the toxic effect and an increase in its anti-cancer function. Also, a patient who was critically down with lymphosarcoma was revived with the aid of DMSO treatment alongside his chemotherapy. Having heard of the great impact of DMSO, the patient requested the possibility of being treated with DMSO solution from his doctor, which the doctor approved even though he (the doctor) wasn't sure of what the outcome might be. The doctor administered the intravenous slow drip injections using 4mg cyclophosphamide per kg of the patient's body weight melted in 1mg DMSO per kg of the patient's body weight 4 times weekly for a period of 6 weeks. There was a great outcome with the patient feeling much better and healthier than he was before the treatment was administered.

Generally, pains from chemotherapy can be excruciating and fatal to the patients, but with the combination of DMSO to this chemotherapy, there's a reduction in pain, side effects are eliminated, and brings out the positive phase of the chemotherapy. Therefore, with adequate use of DMSO and chemotherapy, cancer patients' survival is certain.

♣ <u>Radiation Therapy for Cancer With DMSO.</u>

Over the years, DMSO has been known for its radioprotective properties. Therefore, it is rational for DMSO to be used as a protective agent when a cancer patient is receiving radiation treatment. This idea spanned from a study carried out on some Russian cervical cancer patients. About 22 patients received topical administration of DMSO solution before the commencement of the radiation treatment while about 30 patients were administered the radiation treatment without the application of DMSO solution.

It was recorded that those who received the DMSO application before the radiation treatment was given didn't experience burn from the radiation effect compared to those who didn't receive the DMSO application. Further studies have shown that not only does DMSO protect against burns and toxicity from radiation treatment, but it also increases the effect of the radiation on the cancer ailment.

Treatment Procedures For Radiation Therapy.

- Inject DMSO solution to the patient once a week

- Drink a teaspoonful of DMSO solution mixed in a glass of juice twice daily

- Apply a lotion containing DMSO solution to the patient's chest region twice daily.

♣ DMSO-Laetrile Therapy For Treating Cancer.

DMSO solution combined with laetrile tablet has over the years been used to treat cancer ailments in diverse ways (intravenous injection; slow drip method or via the push method, intramuscular injection method, oral or simple topical application on the cancer region) across the globe.

Life story:

The DMSO-Laetrile therapy was first administered to an artist who had a melanoma tumor that spread across his body (starting from his shoulder) in California. He was placed on regular slow drip treatment of DMSO-laetrile alongside vitamin C. Also, topical application of the DMSO-laetrile solution was administered on the patient's biggest lump (tumor) that grew on his shoulder. Although the patient later died, however, it was recorded that this large lump reduced drastically in size prior to his death because the ailment was already at its peak before DMSO-laetrile therapy was introduced.

Also, the life story of another patient treated with the DMSO-laetrile therapy was that of a lady with tongue cancer and staphylococcus disease at the point of death. A combination of DMSO-laetrile solution and vitamin C was given to her via the intravenous method. After 3 days of using this treatment, this lady could take in liquid foods, and about 3 months later she began living her normal life, gained weight, and forgot ever getting ill in the first place. However, she continued using the DMSO-laetrile tablet even after recovery to prevent cancer reoccurrence.

Another recent incidence is that of a patient who suffered from prostate cancer and was treated with the DMSO-laetrile slow drip therapy method. Although the patient wasn't concerned about the prostate cancer but the resultant effect of the radiotherapy used in treating the cancer that led to radiation cystitis that brought about continuous heavy bleeding to the patient. He was given 3 drops of DMSO solution with about 25gms of vitamin C together with 6gms of laetrile using the intravenous slow drip treatment method for 5 days in 5 weeks. An oral dosage of 1-teaspoon of DMSO solution mixed with 2 drops of aloe-vera juice was also given alongside the intravenous treatment twice daily. This treatment pattern became the end of the bleeding after two weeks of application, the prostate cancer was cured and he lived a normal life even though he continued with treatment.

Treatment Procedure.

- Give 1gm of DMSO per kg of the patient's body weight with 6gms of laetrile and 25gms of vitamin C every 4-hours daily for a period of 5-weeks. Or take a teaspoonful of DMSO solution in 2 ounces of aloe vera juice 5-days a week, for 2 weeks.

- Orally give one teaspoonful of DMSO solution with laetrile tablets and vitamin C followed by a healthy diet pattern containing natural and raw foods.

CHAPTER 8

DMSO THERAPY FOR TREATING CIRRHOSIS OF THE LIVER.

Cirrhosis of the liver is a permanent scaring that damages the liver and results in disruption of its proper functioning. Several deaths have been recorded from this ailment due to excessive smoking, alcohol intake, poor dieting, and several other factors. The ailment poses no symptoms until severe damage to the liver has taken place. Its most probable symptoms include; nausea, edema (swollen legs, feet, or ankles: though not all edema are result of Cirrhosis), weight loss, jaundice, pale fingernails, and fluid deposits in the abdomen.

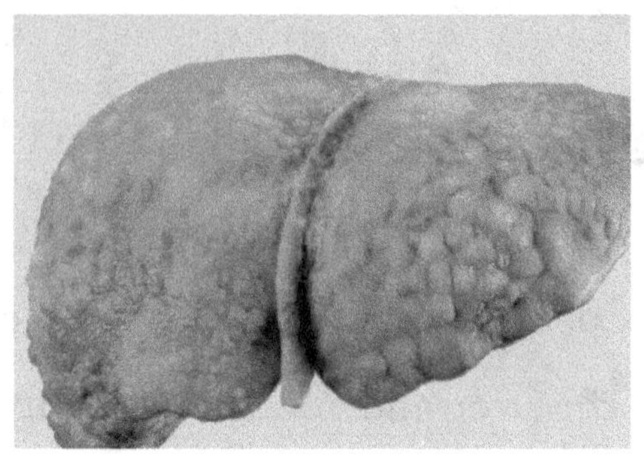

DMSO therapy has over the years proven to be a potent medication for ailments such as this (Liver cirrhosis). It helps to reduce/eradicate virtually all symptoms that accompany the ailment while leading the patient towards total recovery from this sickness and bringing proper functioning to the liver.

Treatment Procedure.

Orally give a teaspoon of DMSO solution mixed with a drop of aloe vera juice twice daily for 6 months.

Note: Every form of habit that poses danger to the liver system must be stopped (never to be returned to) while using DMSO therapy in order to get the desired result.

♣ <u>DMSO Therapy For Diabetes.</u>

Diabetes is a disease that occurs when the pancreas does not produce sufficient insulin (a hormone that regulates blood glucose in the body) or when the body does not properly utilize the insulin produced. There are different types of diabetes; type 1, type 2, and gestational diabetes. Its symptoms range from blurry vision, irregular weight loss, fatigue, and frequent urination (for non-pregnant persons). DMSO has been proven over time to be effective in the treatment of diabetes. From history, DMSO has exhibited amazing ability in treating diabetic neuropathy, a major issue faced by older individuals with a previous history of diabetes ailment. This is often a major problem in older people who have suffered from diabetes for many years. Though using DMSO therapy should not put a stop to the use of insulin (always seek medical advice) some patients have been able to limit the use of insulin by their daily use of DMSO. DMSO helps improve blood supply by expanding the small blood vessels, thereby paving the way for increased blood circulation to the extreme parts of the body. Prevention of diabetes as an ailment should be our ultimate goal hence the advice on adding DMSO solution to every normal medication given to a diabetic patient.

<u>Treatment Procedure.</u>

- <u>Topically:</u> Apply DMSO solution on the patient's toes, feet, and legs twice daily for about 3 weeks.

- <u>Orally:</u> Let the patient drink a teaspoonful of DMSO solution mixed in a cup of juice or water daily after the evening for 3 weeks.

- Engage in regular exercise and proper dieting.

CHAPTER 9
DMSO THERAPY FOR DIGESTIVE PROBLEMS.

Digestive disorders of various types can be very difficult to treat and even more difficult to diagnose. DMSO can significantly moderate the damage to the digestive system particularly when combined with other products such as aloe vera. However, getting the treatment is often not the answer but finding the root cause of the problem/ailment and removing it or limiting it is the major solution/answer.

Life story

A good example involved an eight-year-old girl in Los Angeles who vomited daily after breakfast. She was a recent immigrant to the United States and was staying with an aunt. She was taken to a doctor who said that the girl was suffering from internal bleeding. He referred the girl to a specialist who found that she had a partial blockage caused by a very bad fungus infection. The specialist thought that the infected part of the intestinal tract would probably have to be removed by surgery. Some conventional anti-fungal medications were tried without success. As a last result before surgery, it was decided to try DMSO; which was used for 2 weeks and every symptom of the ailment disappeared. His decision to try DMSO before resorting to surgery saved the girl from major intestinal surgery that could have caused her trouble for the rest of her life.

Treatment Procedure.

Orally: Take ½ teaspoon of DMSO solution mixed with 1 drop of aloe vera diluted in 2 drops of water immediately after breakfast and dinner daily for a period of 2 weeks.

♣ DMSO Therapy For Carpal Tunnel Syndrome. (CTS)

Carpal tunnel syndrome is a numbness, burning, tingling, and painful sensation in the arm that occurs as a result of contraction of the center nerve of the wrist (a nerve that supplies sensations and movements to other parts of the hand). It is one of the common strain injuries often recorded in the workplace. A long-term effect of this ailment can lead to total damage to the hand nerves and weakening of the hands and finger muscles. Several medications for the treatment of this ailment have proven to offer temporary results or even failed in most cases. DMSO with its numerous health benefits is a great remedy for carpal tunnel syndrome because of its anti-inflammatory properties compared to other anti-inflammatory drugs that have harmful side effects after usage. With the proper application of DMSO solution, there will be adequate blood circulation around the affected area and maximum pain reduction to the individual.

Treatment Procedure.

<u>Topical:</u> Topically apply DMSO solution on the arm (from the fingers to the hand down to the upper part of the arm and the elbow) twice daily for 2 weeks.

CHAPTER 10

DMSO THERAPY FOR EAR & HEARING PROBLEMS.

Ear defect affects a large number of the world's population today, particularly children. Ear problems are often treated via puncturing of the eardrum to bring out accumulated pus and relieve pressure on the victim which in most cases, is very painful. However, a combination of DMSO solution and anesthetic drugs makes puncturing the eardrum possible without severe pain.

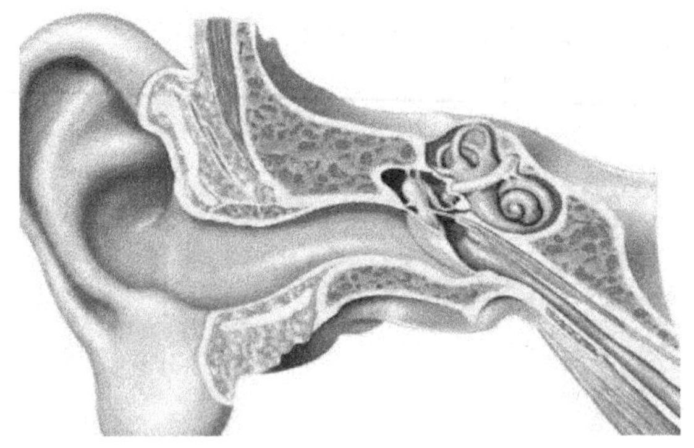

In most cases, individuals with inner ear problems are often treated with a combination of DMSO solution and an antibiotic medication without going through the process of puncturing. The life story of a family of 8 (a man, his wife, and 6 children) whose children suffered ear infections and were later treated with DMSO is a clear description of the potent capacity of DMSO solution as a therapy for hearing/ear problems. This family 6 children suffered ear infections from infancy which further resulted in hearing defects. They were treated with DMSO and there was great relief afterwards.

<u>Treatment Procedure.</u>

- Using an eyedropper, apply 2 drops of 50% concentration of DMSO solution to the affected ear twice daily till the ear heals.

- Topically massage a 90% concentration of DMSO solution on the head of the patient and the neck area close to the affected ear.

♣ <u>DMSO Therapy For Hair And Scalp Problems.</u>

Over the years, both humans (particularly those who went through cancer chemotherapy sessions) and animals (treated with DMSO) with hair loss have been able to stimulate their hair growth with the aid of DMSO solutions with outstanding outcomes.

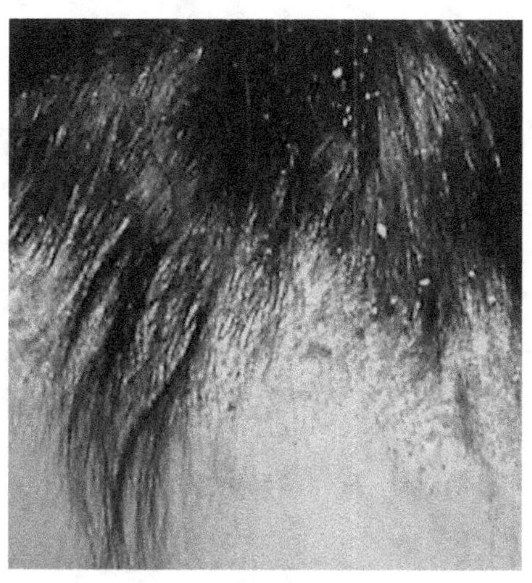

Not only does this solution grow lost hair, but it also enhances the thickness of hair that is already in the area.

Why DMSO Kindle Hair Growth.

DMSO as a vasodilator, helps dilate the smaller capillaries found in the scalp and enhance the supply of blood flow to the hair roots. With this, the needed nutrients for hair growth are sufficiently supplied to the follicles of the hair thereby allowing hair growth to begin. Although the process might be slow for those with male bald hair patterns.

All you need do is topically apply DMSO lotion to the head of the patient daily for at least 6 months.

CHAPTER 11

DMSO THERAPY FOR FUNGUS INFECTIONS.

DMSO has a proven track of effectiveness in the treatment of infectious fungi alongside other skin-related infections; such as jungle rot (mostly found in the hot moist region), athletic foot disease, acne, etc.

♣ DMSO Therapy For Jungle Foot Infection.

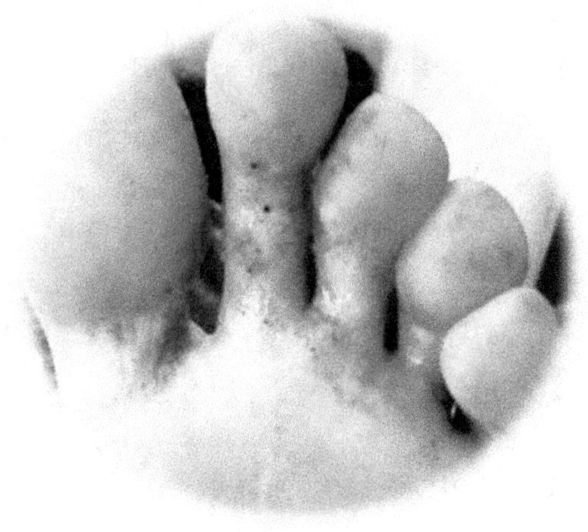

Jungle rot is a serious infection that is found in hot moist areas and is often difficult to treat, once it is contracted. During the Second World War, many soldiers in the South Pacific and Vietnam came down jungle rot because of the moist environment and they were also unable to get proper foot hygiene, their feet were constantly wet while the environment was hot, and were also unable to change their socks or even their jungle boots for several days thereby providing a growth avenue for the infection which eventually spread out to others.

However, with the help of DMSO lotion, one would get "relief" not "cure" from this infectious disease. Though the treatment doesn't give a permanent cure to the ailment, there's immediate relief, and with the constant use of this therapy, one is sure to stay clear of the infection. It is advisable that every veteran have this DMSO lotion as it seems to be one of if not the only best medicine for these infectious fungi.

Treatment Procedure

Apply a skin lotion containing a mixture of DMSO solution and Aloe vera to the affected area daily.

♣ DMSO Therapy For Athlete's Foot Infection.

This is another infectious fungus disease that often responds positively to DMSO treatment. The disease occurs majorly during the summer season and it affects people who always use round-covered shoes that prevent heat from escaping their feet to grant air entry to the feet. Although DMSO treatment works well for this ailment, practicing personal hygiene such as air drying our shoes and socks to properly dry daily helps put these fungi away.

<u>**Treatment Procedure.**</u>

- Get a 60% - 90% concentration of DMSO solution and topically apply it on the feet, toes, and nails twice daily.

- Mix DMSO solution with aloe vera and capsicum pepper and topically apply it on the feet regularly until there's total relief.

- Ensure to always clean your feet, wash socks, and always air-dry shoes.

CHAPTER 12
DMSO THERAPY FOR INFLAMMATORY DISEASE.

Inflammation is one intricate body's response to injuries or destructions of the body tissue due to damage from diseases or fatal injuries. In chronic cases, it is associated with signs such as pains, heat, redness in the affected area, swelling, or total loss of function in the affected area. Conditions like arthritis can result in chronic inflammatory disease. Severe inflammations mostly occur as a result of burns, infections, fatal injuries, or other chronic illnesses. DMSO is a major anti-inflammatory agent as previously mentioned in the course of this book and can help eliminate any trace of inflammatory disease in an individual. It has helped reduce swelling in patients, restore normalcy to localized heat felt by patients, and immediate pain reduction in patients. DMSO helps enhance cortisol efficiency; a steroid hormone produced from the adrenal gland. DMSO also increases the effectiveness of cortisol. Cortisol, which is produced in the adrenal glands serves as the body's natural anti-inflammatory hormone generator. From laboratory research, DMSO has been proven to be very helpful in protecting cells against different harmful agents with or without the presence of cortisol.

Compared to other anti-inflammatory drugs such as steroid drugs (cortisone) and non-steroid anti-inflammatory drugs (NSAIDs) that pose toxic side effects like fluid retention, suppressed immune system, gastrointestinal bleeding, etc. to the patient particularly when used for a long period, DMSO has not only proven to be a potent anti-inflammatory drug, but one with no negative side effects while also addressing other side effects brought on by NSAIDS. DMSO is not just an anti-inflammatory drug, but also one of the major effective free radical scavengers. Rather than cause harm to the gastrointestinal tract, it basically helps to make it healthier.

Treatment Procedure.

- Orally administer a teaspoon of DMSO solution to the patient 4 times daily.

- DMSO solution can also be used alongside dieting and regular exercising for the treatment of arthritis and injuries in patients.

♣ <u>DMSO Therapy For Interstitial Cystitis.</u>

Interstitial Cystitis disease is basically an inflammation of the bladder's inner lining. Its symptoms range from a severe decrease in bladder capacity to bleeding, or even serious scarring to the bladder. Though its symptoms are similar to that of cystitis which is mostly initiated by infectious bacteria and can be treated with antibiotics, but interstitial cystitis disease is not a bacterial infection and doesn't answer to antibiotics treatment. Patients with interstitial cystitis often feel the urge to urinate several times daily with so much pain in their bladder area. This ailment often affects a larger percentage of women compared to men. DMSO was initially approved majorly to treat interstitial cystitis in the 1970s by the FDA because there was no actual treatment remedy for this ailment. As time went by, DMSO became a generally accepted treatment remedy for this disease following its approval by the FDA.

Treatment Procedure.

Two treatment methods are basically used to treat this ailment;

- **Catheter Instilling Method:** this method involves instilling the DMSO into the patient's bladder directly twice weekly. However, some patients complain of severe pains whilst on this treatment method. If this is the case, the second method becomes the best option.

- **Oral method:** Mix a teaspoon of DMSO solution into a glass of water or juice and give it to the patient to drink twice daily.

Also, you can decide to use both treatment methods for a patient; First, begin with the installation method for some time and finish up with the oral method.

♣ <u>DMSO Therapy for Lupus.</u>

Lupus is an inflammation that shows different symptoms in patients (its symptoms differ in individual patients). It can appear in the form of skin rash, joint pains, fatigue, or even fever. In severe cases, it can cause damage to the victim's internal organs, particularly the kidney. A worst case of Lupus infection can result in total immobility to the victim for a while before recovery. DMSO as an alternative medicine has shown itself to be a very potent therapy in the treatment of several ailments including lupus. Though it doesn't outrightly bring a permanent cure to lupus disease, but brings about maximum reduction to its symptoms thereby giving the patient relief from pains associated with the disease.

Treatment Procedure.

- **Intravenous:** Weekly inject DMSO solution on the patient alongside vitamins

- **Topically:** Rub any lotion with DMSO solution in its content to the affected joints daily.

♣ Multiple Sclerosis.

This is an inflammatory disease that causes damage to the myelin sheaths surrounding the brain and spinal cord region and further results in scarring or demyelination. One of the major consequences of this disease is the reduction of the nerve cells' ability to effectively communicate amongst themselves. This disease (Multiple Sclerosis) is of two types generally; the progressive form and the remitting form. The progressive form disables and kills the patient quickly compared to the remitting form which gives room for recovery before outright damage is done to the myelin sheath. Patients with remitting forms of multiple sclerosis have higher chances of living longer compared to those with the progressive form.

<u>Treatment Procedure.</u>

- Give the patient a DMSO intramuscular injection two times daily per week.
- Orally give a teaspoonful of DMSO solution mixed in a glass of water to the patient to drink daily.
- Topically massage the patient's arms and feet with a lotion containing DMSO solution daily.

Follow the above treatment pattern till there's total recovery.

CHAPTER 13

DMSO THERAPY AS A PROTECTION AGAINST RADIATION DAMAGE.

Over the years, DMSO has helped protect individuals from radioactive toxic effects like radiation burns with the aid of its radio-protective properties. Radiation emits free radicals that cause damage to cells in the entire body system. These radicals make the cells age swiftly and also further alter the cell systems resulting in cancer, natal defects, or even other severe diseases.

Several studies have revealed the relevance of DMSO protective abilities on cervical cancer patients who were treated with radiation therapy alongside DMSO. With the aid of DMSO, these patients were protected from radiation burns and other radioactive toxic effects.

<u>Treatment Procedure.</u>

DMSO treatment protocols for radiation vary from individual to individual depending on the case being addressed. It can be given orally, intravenously (injection), or topically (applying it on the skin) though the three methods can be used on a patient. DMSO therapy should be administered to those with massive exposure to radiation.

- Administering a high dosage of this medicine (DMSO) is advisable for those with major radiation exposure considered to be threatening to life particularly those working with power plants. About 5gm per kg of the victim's body weight should be given on the first day within 24-hour intervals and remove the victim from the source of radiation also. Those working with nuclear power plants were advised to be moved 100 miles away from the site of the incident. Reduce the dosage after the first dose to 1gm per kg of the victim's body weight.

- **<u>For Pregnant Women:</u>** Protecting the pregnant mother from radiation is very important as the radiation has the potential to cause deformity in the unborn child, blood cancer, or other severe health conditions. Topically apply an 80%-90% concentration of DMSO solution all over the person's (pregnant woman) body; apply 60%-70% DMSO concentration on the face region. *Note...watch out for possible reaction or adaptability of the patient to this treatment.*

- For patients with radiation burns, a lotion that has 50% DMSO concentration and aloe vera in its content should be applied. Clean the skin off any alcohol substance before applying DMSO solution on the skin twice or thrice daily.

- **<u>For Oral Treatment:</u>** Mix a 20% concentration of DMSO solution in a glass of juice or water and drink a glass after eating daily.

For several years, DMSO has helped treat ailments of all kinds, it has been well known to be one, if not the safest medication out there. Despite its wide usage by many people, there have not been any recorded cases where it had any negative effect aside from its garlic-like odor that fades away within a few minutes.

CHAPTER 14
DMSO THERAPY FOR RESPIRATORY PROBLEMS.

Respiratory problems have been one major challenge that affects young infants (bronchiolitis) as well as aged persons in the society today. This ailment can be deadly in severe cases. However, with the help of DMSO in combination with other antibiotic products and anti-inflammatory medications, one is sure to get relief from this disease. Studies carried out on children with severe respiratory problems showed the positive effect of combining DMSO with the regular conventional treatment regime. These babies were grouped into two categories (Groups A and B). Group A was treated with antibiotics, oxygen, and a steam tent (a waterproof cotton cover) while Group B was treated the same way with the addition of anti-inflammatory drugs and DMSO-containing aerosol spray. From the studies, those who received DMSO treatment had faster recovery compared to those babies who were treated without DMSO. Also, the babies that received DMSO treatment no longer needed the use of a steam tent as the DMSO spray used, helped reduce their inflammation and stickiness in their lungs, and further helped them cough out easily and enhance their breathing capacity.

Treatment Procedure.

Using a tracheal cannula, give the patient 1ml of DMSO solution spray daily. There may be intense coughing and brief choking at first after applying this treatment, but it will normalize after some minutes.

♣ DMSO Therapy For Asthmatic Condition.

Asthma is an inflammation of the bronchial tubes. It is a common illness in children though it is not limited to children alone but cuts across all ages. In acute cases, asthma can result in breathing difficulty that leads to the death of a patient due to lack of adequate oxygen supply. Reducing activities that trigger the attack and inhaling are the major medications for this ailment. Cortisone is often used but the long-term usage of this drug can pose negative side effects to the patient. With the advent of DMSO, positive results without any side effects have been recorded over the years.

<u>**Treatment Procedure.**</u>

Diverse treatment procedures can be applied in the use of DMSO solution solely or when combined with other medications to treat asthma;

- <u>**Topically:**</u> Apply a lotion with aloe vera juice, eucalyptus oil, and DMSO solution in its content on the chest, nose, and forehead of the patient every night before going to bed.
- Always keep the body hydrated with water.
- Avoid things or activities that trigger asthmatic attacks.

Note...other medications in use before DMSO should not be stopped immediately but should be stopped gradually with doctors' supervision till total recovery is achieved.

CHAPTER 15

DMSO THERAPY FOR SKIN DISEASE.

♣ DMSO Therapy For Scleroderma.

Scleroderma also known as system sclerosis is a rare condition that thickens the skin and other tissues of the body. It destroys healthy tissues and changes the skin texture while affecting other organs of the body negatively.

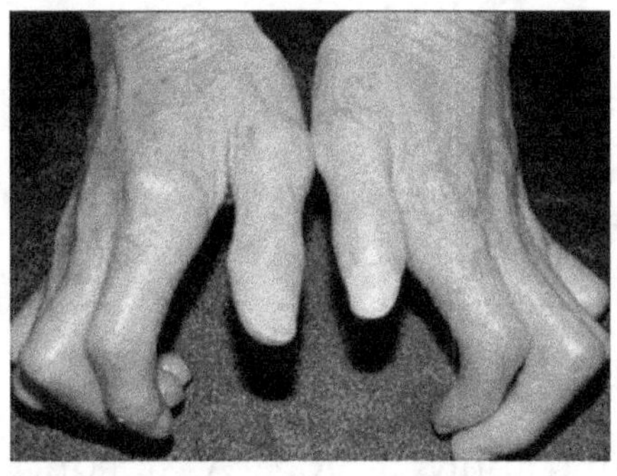

Its cause is unknown hence getting conventional treatment has oftentimes proven abortive. This disease mostly affects people of ages 25-45 years group. The disease progression varies from individual to individual (it can affect only the fingers in some patients while for others, it spreads across).

Life story

A major study on scleroderma was carried out in the early 60s at a clinic in Ohio on about 43 patients ages 1 to 25 years. These patients were treated with DMSO solution for a period of 3 months and observable positive changes were recorded at the end of the treatment.

Treatment Procedure.

- Topically apply a 30%-90% concentration of DMSO solution over the patient's entire body, hands, feet, and legs twice daily for 3 to 5 months

- Orally drink a teaspoonful of DMSO solution mixed in a glass of juice twice daily.

- Engage in regular exercise; walk a distance.

- Get a good diet plan; eat more raw fruits and vegetables. Also, avoid foods that contain processed sugar.

♣ <u>DMSO Therapy For Shingles & Herpes.</u>

Shingles is a viral disease that causes painful rash which forms blisters on the skin. It is caused by varicella-zoster; a virus that causes chickenpox. It is symptoms range from chills, headache, fever, stomach upset, and other symptoms that appear some days later such as body itching, burning sensation in the affected area, skin redness, fluid-filled blisters that break open after some time, etc.

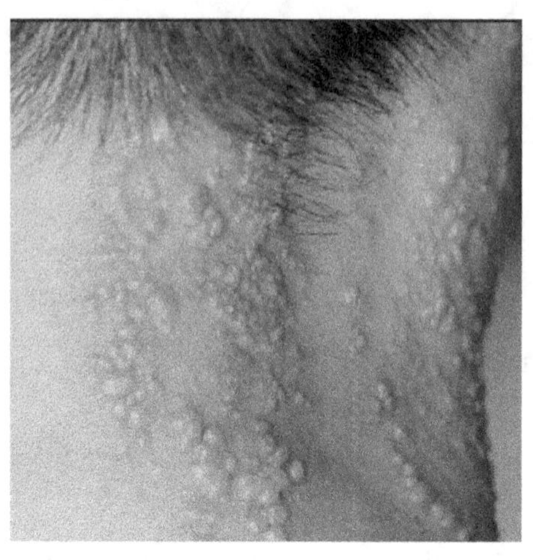

This disease (shingles) usually lasts for a few weeks till total recovery but if it attacks the face region, it has the possibility of getting into the eyes and causing blindness to its victim in severe cases. Most times after the sores fade off, there can lasting pain in the affected areas (post-herpetic neuralgia) which can be excruciating. Preventing this post-herpetic neuralgia is one major thing to do in treating shingles infection and this is done by early treatment of the infection. With the help of

DMSO, a positive solution to this viral infection has been achieved over time. The use of DMSO solely or a combination of DMSO solution with other anti-inflammatory and anti-viral drugs has helped obtain an absolute cure to this ailment.

Treatment Procedure.

There are different treatment procedures when it comes to the use of DMSO therapy in the treatment of shingles infection. Whichever method you choose, is sure to give you your desired result.

- Get a DMSO spray mixed with anti-viral and anti-inflammatory drugs and spray on the affected skin twice daily.

- Apply a 50%-90% concentration of DMSO solution on the affected skin daily. You can also combine DMSO of this same quantity with dexamethasone (a corticosteroid used for treating skin inflammation) and apply it.

- For herpes zoster and herpes simplex infection, you can combine DMSO solution with lysine (an essential amino acid that serves as a building block of protein in the body that helps to restrict the growth of the herpes virus). You can take 2500mg of lysine alongside a teaspoonful of DMSO solution mixed in juice or water orally while topically applying a 50% to 90% concentration of DMSO solution on the affected skin 3 times daily.

Note: To get the best of these treatments, ensure to begin the treatment early enough.

CHAPTER 16

DMSO THERAPY FOR SPINAL CORD INJURIES.

Treating Serious back injuries particularly those that involve the spinal cords is often very difficult, especially with conventional methods of treatment. It majorly occurs as a result of motor accidents, sports injuries, industrial accidents, or other severe trauma incidents.

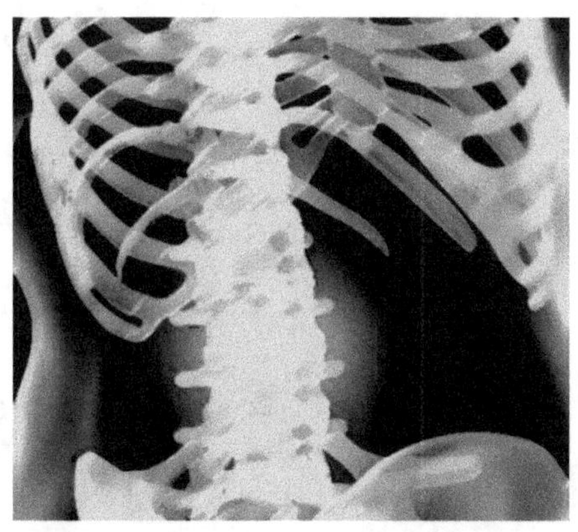

Its level of damage to the individual is usually very difficult to detect until after some time when mobility becomes difficult. One major thing that occurs during spinal cord injury is a decrease in oxygen and blood supply around the body system due to constriction of the body's blood vessels and if there's not adequate or immediate treatment, the tissues of the body can begin to swell further leading to temporal or permanent paralysis.

However, with the aid of DMSO and its unique properties as a free radical scavenger, treating this ailment has been made very easy. With DMSO swellings reduced, there's an increase in blood flow and oxygen supply around the injury site. The intravenous slow drip method of DMSO treatment is often the most effective treatment method for spinal cord injuries. This will help enhance the volume of blood flow in the affected area. The topical and oral method of treatment serves as a follow-up on the intravenous method.

Treatment Procedure.

- Give DMSO intravenous slow drip to the victim immediately after the accident

- Topically massage a DMSO lotion on the affected area twice daily.

- Orally give the patient a teaspoonful of DMSO solution mixed in a glass of water or juice to drink.

♣ DMSO Therapy for Stroke.

DMSO has several amazing healing properties that make it a vital medication in the treatment of any brain-related problems. As such, it should be a sought-after drug in the treatment of stroke patients because of its ability to easily penetrate the blood-brain barrier; a protective layer that exists between the circulating blood and the brain system. DMSO has over the years proven to be an excellent treatment for strokes. With DMSO, excess accumulated fluids that occur in the brain as a result of damage caused by the stroke are removed thereby reducing the pressure to the brain and causing less damage to the brain as well. DMSO helps other blood vessels in the body system do the work of any damaged blood vessels and possibly save the stroke victim's life. It protects the nerve cells from further disruption that follows stroke injury. With the proper and immediate use of DMSO, victims of stroke lives can actually be saved. DMSO should be made available in ambulances to be topically applied to stroke victims while being transported to the hospital with adequate training on how to use this product before further treatments are given. Immediate treatment is needed irrespective of the severity of the injury as delayed treatment might result in permanent brain damage or even death in worst cases.

Treatment Procedure.

- Topically massage DMSO solution on the head of the victim within a few minutes of the incident and twice daily.

- An intramuscular injection of DMSO should be given to the victim a few hours after the stroke incident for the next 2 weeks.

- Two doses of a teaspoonful of DMSO solution mixed in a glass of water or juice should be given to the patient to drink daily.

CHAPTER 17

DMSO THERAPY FOR TOOTH & GUM DISEASE (PERIODONTAL DISEASE).

It is a disease that affects the supporting structure of the teeth; the gum, the teeth bone supporting tissue, and the periodontal brain resulting in gingivitis in its early stage. An inflammation of the gum.

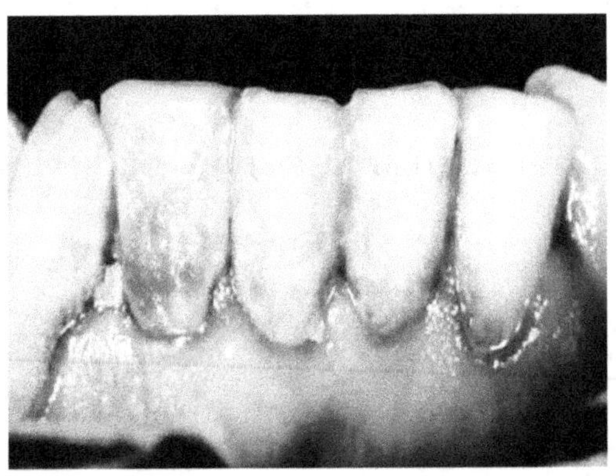

This disease is one major cause of tooth loss in aged people across the globe today. Periodontal disease often occurs as a result of poor oral hygiene and excessive intake of sugar-containing foods. Bacteria feed on particles of these foods, form plaque in the gum, and cause swelling and bleeding to the affected gums. These bacteria eliminate waste, dispose of fecal matter on the teeth and gums, and build up a foul smell in the person's mouth. Without proper treatment, these plagues gradually spread to the core layer of the teeth and bone leading to severe damage to the individual's teeth (periodontitis). At this point, the teeth become loosed and may begin to fall off in the worst cases when treatment is not applied. With the use of DMSO to regularly brush the teeth, these bacteria are greatly reduced, pains reduced, bleeding stopped, loosed teeth get tighter, and normalcy restored to the mouth.

<u>Treatment Procedure.</u>

- Apply a 30% concentration of DMSO compression on the affected teeth for about 10 minutes daily for 7-10 days.

- Use a 50% concentration of DMSO solution to wash your mouth daily.

- **For Extracted Teeth:** topically apply DMSO solution to the jaw surface or cheek close to the extracted site.

CONCLUSION.

Conclusively, DMSO has shown to be among the safest and most important products ever used for the relief of human pains and suffering either solely or in combination with other medications. Its safety to humans has been proven over the years with no contraindications. No toxic reaction case has been recorded from its use by individuals across the globe over the years. DMSO is a healing agent that should be made known to all health care providers at any level with adequate training and guides on how to use this amazing healing agent.

Most times, health practitioners may find it difficult to discover the root cause of some ailments, some ailments may display vague symptoms and inconclusive tests. With this situation at hand, DMSO becomes a useful medicinal option. The possibility of harming anyone is very minimal. Most times, carrying out a double-blind experiment is usually difficult because of its garlic-like odor but patients can be grouped into two categories (treat some groups with DMSO and other groups get treated without DMSO) to get the desired report.

THE END.

www.ingramcontent.com/pod-product-compliance
Lightning Source LLC
Chambersburg PA
CBHW070912260726
48661CB00004B/1708